SPINE SURGERY RECOVERY

How to Prepare Your Home and Take Care of Yourself to Minimize Pain and Stress

SANDRA JOINES

Contents

Why Should I Read This Book?

According to the Agency for Healthcare Research and Quality, there are approximately 500,000 low back surgeries performed each year in the United States. That sounds like an awful lot of spine surgeries, making your procedure no different from thousands of others. But, your surgery will be unique to you and probably will be the only surgery about which you will care.

This book is not about me or my surgery. It is about you and what you can learn from my experiences to help make your recovery less painful and less stressful. This book will show you how to make simple, inexpensive changes to your home that will allow you to navigate through your recovery more conveniently and with less difficulty. It is about how you can easily implement and make the best of all instructions that will be provided to you by healthcare professionals and turn your *what-to-do's* into *how-to-do's.*

1

It will also assist your caregivers in understanding your needs and how to best help you move through the difficult recovery period.

Think about it this way. Your surgeon, the person who conducts the spine class you may be privileged to attend, and the hospital will provide you with instructions telling you what you can and cannot do after surgery. These instructions, however, do not explain *how to do* or *how not to do* these things.

This is where I come in. I will cover many of the requirements listed in your instructions and share with you through my experiences simple, affordable solutions, written in easy, down-to-earth words.

I am not an expert in any area of the medical profession and will be the first person to tell you to **always consult with your medical professionals for instructions and advice.** I have become an expert, however, at how to prepare your home and take care of yourself to make your recovery period less painful and less stressful.

The mere thought of spine surgery can be extremely frightening and overwhelming. Giving someone you hardly know complete access to your body and basically control of your life are huge decisions. Spine surgery is definitely an undertaking that should not be taken lightly and a decision that should be well contemplated.

Unless you have life-threatening issues or pain so intense that immediate surgery is required, the choice for surgery is up to you. You have to consider what effect your spine condition is having on your life. Are the limitations keeping you from doing the things you enjoy most? Are you no longer able to take care of your daily personal needs? Can you no longer tie your shoes? Are you unable to walk? Can you no longer lift your child or grandchild? Has your pain escalated to the point where it is unbearable and it is affecting your quality of life to a degree where it is no longer acceptable to continue the way you are?

Perhaps you are in the earlier stages of spine issues where surgery could possibly slow down continued progression, or maybe your need for surgery is required due to an accident. Possibly you qualify for a minimally-invasive procedure. Lucky you! Most of us wish we were fortunate enough to have our issues corrected with this type of surgery.

What I am going to share with you is not specific to the type of procedure you are facing, how many levels of your spine are involved, or which vertebrae will be affected. Anyone having spine surgery will have challenges and can benefit from my recovery experiences as a spine surgery patient.

Remember, I am not offering medical advice. Always consult your surgeon, primary care physician, or any medical professional who has been assigned to you for advice. Follow their instructions.

As I said before, I am an expert at being a spine surgery patient who has survived her recovery journey. I will share with you the actions I took to be a part of the decisions for medical care and to stay in control of my body.

If you follow only a few of the suggestions I have provided for preparing yourself and your home for your recovery period, I promise that your life after surgery will be considerably less painful and less stressful. You will also be more content knowing that you will not have to be completely dependent on your caregivers for many of your personal needs during your spine surgery recovery.

Heading Home and Hunkering Down

You have made it through the surgery and survived your hospital stay, and now it is time to go home and settle in. The process of being discharged from the hospital and getting home sounds simple enough: sign the discharge papers, listen as the nurse reviews the instructions you are required to follow, ride to the car in a wheelchair, get into the automobile, and be driven home.

Not so easy. In my case, a considerably long time passed after a nurse informed me that I was going to be discharged from the hospital before the proper paperwork was processed and I was being wheeled out of the hospital main entrance by a friendly woman who liked to talk.

Upon reaching the car my husband had driven into the patient pickup area, the friendly woman opened the car door and looked at me. I looked at her. No one had talked to me about how to get into a vehicle, and I didn't remember seeing any instructions in the ton of paperwork I had been provided.

The friendly woman held up her index finger, as if to say *just a moment*, ran back into the hospital, and returned with a plastic bag, which she placed on the seat of the car to help me slide in more easily.

She instructed me to stand up from the wheelchair, take a few steps to the car, turn, and back up to the seat. Easy enough, right? But, there was this thing called pain, and as I backed to the seat, carefully lowering myself while bracing my hands against the door frame, my head hit the top of the frame.

It doesn't seem like a problem. Right? Simply duck my head and get on in. As it turned out, however, ducking my head would have led to bending and twisting my back. It took several tries to figure out how to maneuver my body to get my head under the frame without bending or twisting.

Once my head and my body were both in the car, the plastic moved easily with me as I lifted my legs and turned my entire body at one time to face forward. I will further discuss the techniques of getting into and out of an automobile in Chapter Fifteen.

I share this experience to show you how complicated simple things can be after spine surgery. As much as I had prepared for my recovery, it never once occurred to me that not only should I have practiced, prior to surgery, how to get in and out of a car without twisting or turning, but also how to duck my head under the door frame without engaging my body in motions that were painful as well as not allowed.

The painful ordeal of getting into the car increased my readiness to be home and in my own bed. I could not wait for some peaceful sleeping and good food.

Upon arriving home, I tried to reverse the moves I had made to get into the car at the hospital and slowly manipulated myself out of the car. I soon discovered that even the simple process of walking to the door using a walker was exhausting and painful.

Although there were only two steps leading into my home, I found I needed help in order to keep my balance while I lifted my foot to step up. Yes, it hurt!

We should have anticipated the need for installing a handrail on the door frame, but we had spent so much time analyzing the inside of our home, we completely let the outside slip.

This is another example of how simple things never cross our minds until there is a need. Having taken care of this easy fix in advance would have spared me some inconvenience and pain and relieved my husband from feeling some concern for not thinking of it in advance.

It had been a struggle getting in and out of the car and climbing the two steps to get into my home, and I wanted nothing more than to go to my bed and rest. When I got to the foot of the stairs leading to the second floor, I looked up and sighed. The fourteen stairs might as well have been four hundred.

With the help of my husband and daughter, I slowly climbed the first seven stairs, making sure I did not bend forward. I rested at the landing for a few seconds before tackling the next seven. After five more steps I heard loud noises echoing throughout the house. It took a few seconds more to realize the cries were coming from me. I knew at that moment that I never wanted to go back down those stairs or see stairs ever again in my life. EVER.

I have no words of wisdom as to how to climb stairs right after you have surgery. What I can say is to be prepared for pain and difficulty and have someone by your side. Then simply stay away from stairs until your body is more willing and able to accommodate them.

Not long after climbing the stairs and taking pain medication, my two caregivers had me out of my clothes, into my own comfy nightgown, and sitting on the side of the bed ready to be tucked away between soft sheets that smelled like spring flowers. To be perfectly honest, I think my screaming on the stairs had them a little rattled.

I sat there, like a mushroom, thinking that lying down would be a piece of cake because I had practiced the log roll over and over in this bed before surgery. This technique was designed to allow the body in a position that protects the spine from twisting when getting into and out of the bed.

Even though there was a considerable difference in practicing a maneuver before my body was riddled with pain and when every movement made me want to cry out, surely it had to be a lot easier than it was in the narrow hospital bed with IV and oxygen tubes connected to me. Right?

After backing to the bed until my legs touched it and I was carefully sitting down, I extended my left hand in a fluid movement as if I were reaching out for a long, graceful stroke in a warm ocean. My body followed as if it was an extension of my arm, as it was supposed to do. Lying on my side, with my knees bent up towards my chest and with my feet still in contact with the bed, I then moved the extended arm to my chest and, along with my other arm, hugged my body. This position allowed me to roll my whole body onto my back, moving my head, shoulders, hips, and knees all at the same time, without bending or twisting - like rolling a log.

It was painful and nowhere near as easy as it was when I practiced, but I do feel that working on it before surgery made it familiar, a little less painful, and whole lot less stressful.

The pain meds began to kick in, and although the room seemed to spin, creatures began to creep out of the walls, and I said ridiculous things to my family members, I was home. I was with family, and these demons were mine. All was good.

In the next chapter let's explore your limitations regarding bending, lifting, and twisting.

TIPS & ACTION ITEMS

- Practice getting in and out of an automobile using a plastic bag on the seat
- Install handrails at entrances
- Practice log rolling in and out of bed

No BLT!

This has nothing to do with a delicious bacon, lettuce, and tomato sandwich. **NO BLT** with regard to spine surgery recovery means **no bending, lifting, or twisting.** Preventing your body from doing these three things is crucial to your successful healing. This one term will be stressed to you over and over by almost every medical professional with whom you come in contact.

You have read in the previous chapter how I practiced **NO BLT** when I got in and out of the car, when I climbed stairs, and when I log rolled into bed.

My surgeon was the first to bring up the term **NO BLT** during a pre-surgery appointment. I am sure that my raised eyebrows were a sure sign that I had no idea what he meant. But, wait!

A paper clip appeared in his hand. A paper clip, he said, can be thrown against a wall over and over and nothing happens. But, he said, if you take the clip and bend it repeatedly, it eventually breaks.

This broken clip demonstrated that it is the repetition of the bending movement that is the biggest concern. The surgeon told me that movement of the plate and screws caused by this bending and twisting could present a need for him to reopen my back, remove the hardware, and then replace it. OH NO! **NO BLT** for me. For sure. I had this.

Being back home in my own environment and with my husband and daughter as caregivers was precisely what the doctor ordered, so to speak, and I managed to get in and out of the car, climb stairs, and log roll into bed without bending, lifting, or twisting.

In the next chapter, I would like to discuss how practical adjustments and additions to my home helped me during spine surgery recovery and how these simple steps will help you.

TIPS & ACTION ITEMS

- Understanding the reasons for **NO BLT**
- Understanding complications for not following **NO BLT**

Preparing the Kitchen and Living Room

You are home from the hospital and have managed to succeed at getting in and out of the car, climbing stairs, and log rolling into bed. Sure, you felt pain and you will continue to do so for quite a while. But, you have learned how following the rules of **NO BLT** will not only prevent a certain amount of pain, but also will help you heal more successfully during spine surgery recovery.

Perhaps this is a good time to address housecleaning. Since you will not be able to attend to household chores for a while, make arrangements before surgery to have someone available to clean your home.

After surgery, your physical restrictions will cause you much anxiety, and you will soon feel as if you are inconveniencing your caregivers when you have to constantly ask for their assistance. There are a few simple adjustments you can make before your surgery that will help you be more independent. Let's take a look at what you can do in your kitchen and living room.

Kitchen

Think about the items you frequently use and make sure they are stored where you can reach them without bending or standing on your tippy toes. For instance, if your cereal is on a top shelf, move it to a lower shelf. If the pots and pans you use often are housed in your lower cabinet, you will not be able to reach them without assistance. Move them to an upper shelf where you can access them easily. The things you use less frequently can be stored in the places you cannot reach, and you can ask for assistance when you need any of them.

The same applies with your refrigerator. Move the shelves around to make more room for the items you use frequently to be conveniently located within your reaching capability. If you have the freezer-on-top refrigerator, it will be easy for you to access frozen foods and ice. However, vegetable drawers located at the bottom will be difficult for you to reach until you master the squatting-with-**NO-BLT** technique.

You cannot do without a reacher or grabber device to assist you in your kitchen. They come in lengths from 26 to 32 inches and in lightweight aluminum, plastic, and more durable materials designed to pick up heavier items. I would suggest you choose ones with serrated jaws and flexible foam rubber tips that efficiently conform to the contours of any object. Many of the trigger-action handles are ergonomically designed for less stress on your hand and fingers.

I also recommend having a second reacher in the kitchen. Why? If you were to drop your reacher, how would you pick it up?

If you have a conventional oven, being able to maneuver your body into a position that allows you to access the oven with **NO BLT** will be difficult. It will be mandatory to have someone help you until your surgeon releases you from your bending and twisting limitations. The same applies with loading and unloading a dishwasher.

NOTE: It is a good idea to remove throw rugs from the floor, and also remember that many items in a kitchen weigh more than you think. Following the weight guidelines for lifting that your surgeon provided you is essential to your proper healing.

Living Room

Again, remove all throw rugs and make sure a reacher is within easy access. While we are discussing removing items, make sure your caregivers keep the walkways clear of clutter. Small children (or grown children) love to leave a trail of toys, backpacks, and shoes.

Most living room furniture is nice and cozy, but not suitable for sitting after back surgery. Make sure there is a straight-back chair for your use. It might not be as comfortable as you would like, but it will meet the requirements your back needs during the healing process.

If there are items you use that are not within easy reach, move them where they can easily be accessed without your breaking the bending, lifting, and twisting rule. The process of preparing your living and kitchen areas to make your spine surgery recovery easier is simply a common-sense approach. Look over every area of the room and determine what can be done to make it safe and accommodating. Do the same for your bedroom, which we will discuss in the next chapter.

TIPS & ACTION ITEMS

- Arrange for housecleaning

- Keep two reachers within easy reach

- Move frequently-used items in your kitchen cabinets to shelves that are easily within your reach

- Arrange your refrigerator shelves to allow easy access to frequently-used items

- Understand using the oven and loading/unloading the dishwasher will break the **NO BLT** rule

- Remove throw rugs from the kitchen and living area floors

- Store frequently-used items in your living room where you can easily reach them

- Make sure you have a straight-back chair

- Keep walkways free of clutter

Preparing
the Nest

After listening to suggestions from my surgeon, primary care physician, and the nurses who conducted the spine class I attended, I realized more than ever that there were countless home adjustments that could be implemented to better prepare myself and my bedroom for the spine surgery recovery period.

With this in mind, my husband and I carefully looked over the areas where I would spend the majority of time after returning home from the hospital. As we contemplated the bedroom and bathroom, it became apparent that not only did these rooms need to be comfortable, they also needed to provide an atmosphere where I felt safe and secure, a peaceful place where I could relax, a place away from lots of activity so that I could avoid unpleasant sounds, and a place where everything I needed on a daily basis would be at my fingertips: a *nest*.

Together we began a quest to determine what my needs would be, analyze the space, and do whatever was necessary to make my bedroom this perfect nest I was imagining.

Bed

As I was practicing getting in and out of bed using the *log-roll procedure*, it was apparent that the bed was too high. Fortunately, we were able to switch out the mattress and box springs with those from a bed in the guest room. The height of the bed then hit me above my knees and below my bottom, which turned out to be the perfect height for backing up to and lowering my body to a sitting position.

Next, the fancy comforter and the mounds of decorative pillows on the bed were stored away. This left white sheets and a white down alternative comforter. Why all white? *Because white can be bleached, and bleach kills bacteria.* An alternative down comforter is an excellent choice for a cover during winter or summer and can be easily laundered.

Pillows

I don't know about you, but having chronic back pain for years has taught me the art of using pillows, lots of pillows. I have consistently used one under my knees when lying on my back, one between my knees when on my side, one under my shoulder or arm, and a flat one, sometimes a fluffier one, under my neck. You get the picture. So we made sure I had a sufficient number of pillows to accommodate my body's addiction.

Neck Wrap

After returning home from the hospital, I also experienced pain in my neck that lasted a good three weeks or more. I do not know what they did to me while I was in surgery, but I think a big Mack truck was somewhere in the picture.

My daughter is a problem solver. She arrived one afternoon holding a little white lamb. It turned out that the stuffed animal was an aromatherapy neck wrap filled with rice, cinnamon, cloves, and eucalyptus. The neck wrap can be heated in a microwave or cooled in the freezer to be used for a heating or cooling pad. I used the lamb constantly during the first few weeks, and still love to feel its warmth under my neck, as well as smell its spicy aroma.

Look for Spa Comforts Hot and Cold Aromatherapy Neck Wrap, Merry Little Lamb. It also comes in a dog, cat, polar bear, leopard, etc., and can be purchased on Amazon for $19-$25.

Bed Tray

Before surgery when my husband and I were preparing my nest, I lay in the bed and attempted to reach the nightstand located close by, with pain and limited motion in mind. In order to reach anything on top of the nightstand without twisting or bending, I was forced to roll on my side. This led me to think about post-surgery pain and stiffness and how difficult it would be for me to roll over on my side and extend my arm each time I needed an item. Remember, **NO BLT**.

It was an easy fix for my husband. He came up with the idea of taking a wooden kitchen tray and transforming it into a bed tray. With the tray conveniently located next to me, I was able to easily pull it to me and then push it back to the side of the bed out of my way. The one-inch sides prevented items from rolling off while it was being moved back and forth. The cell phone and iPad chargers were plugged into an outlet located behind the bed, and the wires were secured around the handle of the tray. This simple step allowed the phone and iPad to remain on the tray, within my reach, while they were being charged.

I placed items such as glasses, a small note pad and pen, lip balm, body lotion, hand sanitizer, tissues, an Emory board, and a container of face/hand wipes on the tray. It was an incredible whatever-I-needed tray, right there beside me, providing easy access with **NO BLT**.

This simple idea worked remarkably well and cost absolutely nothing. I kept the tray by my side for the three-month period when bending, twisting, and lifting were not allowed. It was easy to pull the tray close and remove what I needed without moving any part of my body other than my arm.

Ceiling Fan

While lying flat on my back in the lowered bed and admiring the handy-dandy convenient tray next to me, I happened to look up at the ceiling fan, which was quietly providing a steady flow of nice cool air. I love the fan on, but have the tendency to adjust the setting throughout the night to accommodate my changing body temperature.

There was no way I could reach the chain while lying in the bed, and thinking about the pain associated with log rolling out of the bed each time I wanted to adjust the setting was a little overwhelming. I was not sure even if standing I could reach the chain over the bed without bending or twisting.

I had an epiphany, which seemed a simple fix to me. Of course, everything has a tendency to sound like a simple fix when my husband is involved. He obliged my request and extended the chain to enable me to reach it with my toes. Now, you have to understand that grabbing things monkey-style is nothing new to me.

This was a lifesaver after surgery. Something as simple as lengthening a chain gave me another small slice of independence. While lying in bed on my back, I was able to reach the little knob, secure it between my toes, and give it a gentle pull in order to change the setting on the fan. The best part was I did not have to call my husband to adjust it for me. I think he liked the idea as much as I did. I am sure you are asking, "Why not install a new fan with a remote control?" My answer would be a simple, "Because our solution was less expensive and faster."

Chair

I was advised during the spine surgery class and in my instructions from the surgeon that straight-back chairs would be required. No cushy, comfy ones would be allowed for spine surgery patients. There was no chair of that type living anywhere in our house. To meet this requirement, my husband and I set out on a mission to find three comfortable straight-back chairs (well, as comfortable as a straight-back chair could be) to place throughout the house.

We searched all of the furniture stores, as well as specialty shops, and found nothing that fit me adequately. During a visit to Lowe's, we came across a wicker-type patio chair with a straight back and arms. The chair was fairly comfortable and kept me at what seemed a proper non-slouching position. It was an incredible find at $59. We bought three and found comfortable pillows for the bottoms at a discount store for $14.99 each.

The chairs worked well, and placing a bed pillow behind my back created a buffer between the chair and my tender incision.

Foot Stool

As I was sitting in one of the chairs that had found a home in the corner of my *nest*, my husband noticed that I seemed unable to find a comfortable position for my legs. I certainly couldn't cross them. They sort of dangled.

Remember, my husband is a problem solver. An easy solution to him was providing me with a small foot stool upon which to rest my dangling feet. After disappearing for a while, he returned to the nest with a small stool he had constructed from scraps. It was about sixteen inches wide, seven inches deep, and maybe five inches high. It was a perfect height. I was able to easily push it under the chair and pull it back out with, yes, my feet and **NO BLT.**

Zipping out to a workshop and whipping up a foot stool is not an option for everyone. You might have one somewhere in your home already or might be able to pick one up for a reasonable price to use with your straight-back chair.

Table

I figure by now you have come to the conclusion that my husband is quite an industrious and creative person. He demonstrated these remarkable traits over and over again as he addressed issues such as the fourteen stairs from my nest to the main living level of our home. Considering the difficulty I had climbing the stairs, it was pretty apparent that it would not be probable, during the first few weeks after surgery, for me to be climbing up and down the stairs for meals.

Therefore, creative husband decided I needed a table in the nest. Not any table, mind you, but one that would be exactly the right height when I was sitting in the perfect straight-back chair with my feet resting on the stool. For some reason I ended up with an extra walker, one of those aluminum ones upon whose back legs colorful tennis balls are often placed. On top of this extra walker, my husband secured a piece of board. It became a table.

Having the right material on hand to build a table or having a partner who is capable and willing to do so is not always an option. But, it is an excellent way to save a little money and shows you how easy it is to come up with ideas.

There are other options. You may have a table living around your house that could possibly work well. The table needs to be sturdy enough to be easily moved with your hands and feet without it toppling over. A metal TV tray is not a good choice. It is light and could easily turn over.

A portable laptop table is an excellent choice and reasonably inexpensive. Several styles can be ordered from Amazon. For example, a Seville Classics Mobile Laptop Desk Cart can be purchased for $34.99. It is positioned on wheels that allow you to roll it around until it is conveniently located, and it does not get in the way of your legs. The height can be easily adjusted. Dimensions: 24" W x 16" D x 20.5" to 33" H.

Clothing

When planning a location for your various clothing items, think not only about your convenience, but also the convenience of your caregivers. Choose the clothing you plan to wear during your recovery and hang the pieces in an area of your closet that is easy to access. The same applies to looking through your drawers and moving the items you plan to wear during your recovery to drawers you can easily reach without bending.

Your caregivers will appreciate your clothing being neatly grouped, and you will feel less stress knowing your clothes are nicely organized and easily accessible.

Speaking of clothing! Make it simple during your recovery. Cotton is not the best choice for pajamas and nightgowns. It does not move freely with your body, especially when getting in and out of your bed.

Plain old sweats with an adjustable waist are great to wear around the house, and they will keep your incision happy.

Reachers

These little contraptions are among my favorite things. I can't always use my toes. They can be purchased at the local dollar store for a buck each or from hardware stores for a small amount more. I found the ones at the hardware stores to be a little better built. I previously mentioned that a higher-quality reacher would be better to address heavier and bulkier items in the kitchen, but less expensive ones work quite adequately in the bedroom.

I hung one on my bedpost, and the other found a home leaning against the wall. Again, why two? If I were to drop one, how would I pick it up?

As you can see, it took only a few improvements to my bedroom to make it much more convenient and comfortable during my recovery time. Crawling up on the high bed would have been extremely painful. Likewise, it would have been impossible for me to reach over to my nightstand to grab an item I needed without bending or twisting, or without log rolling out of bed and standing, only to log roll back into the bed, without the handy-dandy bed tray. There is absolutely no way I could have adjusted the ceiling fan settings by myself without the lengthened chain.

We all have our own individual needs based on our preferences, the type of surgery we have, and plain old body differences. I am sure if you look over your bedroom, you will come up with adjustments and/or additions that will make your recovery significantly easier.

Some can be achieved by using items and material you have on hand, others can be purchased with a small amount of money, and a few may cost a little more. Creativity will help you get through your recovery with less pain and less stress!

If you make simple adjustments to your bathroom, you will find fighting your tendencies to bend and twist less of an issue. In the next chapter, we will discuss these adjustments and also steps you can take to make the area safer during your spine surgery recovery.

TIPS & ACTION ITEMS

- Adjust your bed height
- Store away the comforter & decorative pillows
- Replace the above with a white, down alternative comforter
- Purchase white bed linen
- Place lots of pillows on your bed
- Practice using pillows for maximum comfort for your body
- Purchase a neck wrap
- Set up a bed tray
- Lengthen the chain on your ceiling fan if it is located above your bed or replace the fan with one that has a remote control
- Purchase an acceptable straight-back chair or use one you have
- Purchase or build a foot stool
- Purchase or build a laptop/meal table
- Organize your clothing
- Purchase several reachers

Setting Up
The Bathroom

I am fortunate to have a bath that joins my bedroom. However, there are twenty-one long steps from the side of the bed to the toilet. At times, those steps seem like a hundred, and I cannot imagine having to walk even farther down the hall whenever my body demands it and when I am still walking as slowly as a snail crawling through honey.

NOTE: Plan ahead. It takes time to properly log roll out of bed, put on your back brace, secure your walker, walk to the bathroom, and slowly sit. Since surgery can affect your bladder, it is not a bad idea (just in case) to have a package of adult disposable absorbency underwear on hand to get you through those first days

when your body is moving more slowly but your
bladder is moving with more urgency.

Before surgery, my husband and I made some simple
changes that helped considerably with my personal care.
Take a look below. Perhaps some of these ideas might
make things more convenient for you.

Reachers

Here we go again with one of my favorites items. One lives
hanging on the towel rack right by the sink. I have used
this to pick up numerous items that have slipped right out
of my hand and also to reach the inside of the bottom
cabinets to grab that one thing I needed that I failed to
make easily accessible. Would you believe this particular
item will pinch and pick up something as small and flat as
a pill or a straight pin? If your bathroom does not join your
bedroom, I highly recommend following the two-reacher
rule.

Personal Items

Before surgery, I placed the personal items I use every day
or regularly during a week on the bathroom counter. After
carefully assessing their use and my need for them, I
separated them into two groups. The group of items I
could do without were placed in a cabinet, and the second

group found a home in a basket that I placed on the counter, where they would be easily within my reach.

This basket made an excellent storage device for items such as my hair dryer, curling iron, hair products (other than shampoo), cotton face pads, wash cloths (rolled neatly to save room), girl pads, hair clips (clipped to the basket handles), and a hair brush.

The medicine cabinet and under-counter drawers provided excellent storage for smaller items such as meds and makeup.

Speaking of meds, it would be extremely helpful for your caregivers if you prepared a spreadsheet to record the name of the medication, date it was prescribed, number in bottle, purpose, doctor prescribing, dosage strength, frequency, and when to refill it.

This simple spreadsheet will allow your caregivers to keep track of your prescriptions and when to refill them. It will also provide a place for your caregivers to record the time each of your meds was administered and any reactions you have to the meds.

It doesn't matter where you store your own items or in what type of container. The important part is that you put away everything that is not essential and organize the other items that you use regularly in a place that allows you easy access without bending or twisting. This may seem insignificant now, but simple steps like these will cause you less stress when you are in pain and can't bend and reach as you could before surgery.

Note: Ladies, if you are still dealing with the monthly stuff, it is an excellent idea to have pads on hand. You could find it anywhere from difficult to impossible to use tampons.

The last step was to place a bottle of alcohol next to the sink, which will be addressed in Chapter Nine.

After finally completing the steps of properly getting into my bed, shortly after getting home from the hospital (when I was on meds that made me see spiders crawling up and down the wall and made me feel as if the whole room was spinning around) nature called. I log rolled out of bed. It was painful. My husband secured my back brace after helping me stand and gain my balance. It was painful. I gripped the handles of the silver walker and began taking slow steps to the bathroom (21 steps to the toilet). It was painful.

Guess what? The walker was too wide to fit through the door to the bathroom. We never considered this possibility when we were setting up the area before surgery. There was an easy remedy, though. The door was removed from the hinges and stored away.

No matter how much planning we accomplished before surgery, we discovered things that never once crossed our minds; like the door being too narrow for the walker, for instance.

TIPS & ACTION ITEMS

- Have pads and adult disposable absorbency underwear on hand

- Purchase one or two reachers

- Clear unnecessary items from your counter

- Fill a basket or other container with items you use regularly and place it on the counter

- Clear the medicine cabinet and drawers under the counter from unnecessary items

- Prepare a spreadsheet for tracking meds

- Place a bottle of rubbing alcohol on the counter

- Insure your doorways are wide enough for your walker to pass through

- If not, remove the doors from the hinges and store them away

How To's
In the Shower

The shower was a relatively easy area to prepare. I stepped back, considered what I normally used and contemplated the most efficient way to store these items.

A shower caddy was already hanging from the showerhead and would continue to house shampoo, conditioner, liquid soap, and the wonderful antibiotic soap that I would use right before surgery and after returning home.

With the thought in mind that the container of liquid soap was bound to find its way out of my hand and onto the floor of the shower, I took my favorite bar of soap, wrapped it in netting, and secured it to the caddy. (soap-on-a-rope)

On the bottom hooks, I hung two long-handled scrubbies. These can be found at most stores that sell soap and shampoo, for as low as $2.99 for one with a sturdy handle. I do recommend purchasing the sturdy ones with long handles to make it easier to get to those hard-to-reach areas.

Why two? One is green and one is blue. Blue is for bum. I have to give credit to the spine class I attended for the blue-for-bum idea.

The hand-held *showerhead* my husband installed turned out to be a priceless addition. There was no difference in functionality than with a fixed head, but it was convenient to be able to detach it from the mount and take the water to my body instead of moving my body to the water. This showerhead quickly earned the title of my *#2 favorite tool*.

That being said, there were a couple of negative aspects associated with this type of showerhead. First, the water hose connecting the head to the mount had a tendency to swing around and knock shampoo and other items from the caddy.

A caddy with a deep area for storing personal items would be one way to minimize this issue. However, my husband discovered a caddy that was specifically designed to hang from a hand-held showerhead. Amazon sells an InterDesign Forma Ultra Caddy for $37.99.

This caddy has a split down the center to accommodate the water hose and a clip at the bottom to secure the hose when it is not in use. There are two storage compartments on either side to securely house personal items.

Four hooks are located at the bottom of the caddy. They provide the perfect place for the two scrubbies to hang out.

A less expensive approach would be to secure a plastic caddy, which attaches to the tile using suction cups, over to the side and out of the way of the hose. The suction cups do not always adhere to certain types of stone tile, and the caddy tends to slide downwards when heavy shampoo bottles are stored in it.

The second negative issue hit me right in the face, literally. After placing the showerhead back on the mount, the hose twisted and caused the showerhead to move and spray water directly into my face and all over my hair

Even with a couple of negative aspects, a hand-held showerhead was a valuable asset, and kits can be purchased for around fifty bucks or higher. This was an inexpensive investment with a large kick in convenience.

The most logical place to hang a towel was as close to the shower as possible to keep me from having to take extra steps to retrieve it or tempting me to twist. Once again, my crafty husband placed one of those quick-on and quick-off hangers right outside the door of the shower.

For convenience, a shower cap and head wrap were secured on a towel bar located next to the shower.

To prevent slipping on the tile floor, we placed a non-slip rug directly in front of the shower.

After spending time in a hospital, my body craved the feel of warm water and cleanliness. Fortunately, my shower was small with a low lip to step over, which made it convenient and safe to enter and exit. Being able to place my hands against the shower walls helped me maintain good balance.

Many showers are large enough to accommodate a shower chair. Mine was not. Sitting on a shower seat is safer until your balance returns, but stepping over a conventional tub to get to a shower seat can be challenging. You will need more than a person's hand to assist. Installing shower bars could be your best bet.

By all means, place a sturdy, non-slip rubber mat in the bottom of the tub or shower.

Hopefully, the hospital therapist discussed your personal shower setup and recommended what is best for you and your particular situation. **Please follow the advice provided by medical personnel.**

Note: Your walker is not meant to take the place of shower safety bars. Do not use your walker for leverage to enter or exit your bathtub. It can easily slip and cause you to fall.

During the first few days, my daughter helped me into the shower, sprayed me with nice warm water with the hand-held showerhead, and cleaned the clear bandage over the incision and the skin around it with the same antibiotic soap I was required to use before surgery.

It was important to me to be able to take care of my personal needs by myself as soon as I could. It took practice and patience, but soon I was able to squeeze liquid soap onto the long-handled scrubbies and reach most areas of my body without too much difficulty, remembering not to bend or twist.

After a few trial runs, I was able to adequately maintain my balance to dry my back by running the towel down my back while holding the towel with both hands. Standing with my feet spread, I found that I could dry the inside of my legs and my bottom by tossing the towel between my legs, catching it between my thighs, and slowly pulling it back. The areas I could not reach had to depend on the old drip-dry method.

We talked about showering, drying off, and how my daughter cleansed over the bandaged incision area during my spine surgery recovery. Now let's discuss how my husband and daughter took care of my incision by changing the bandage every day until the stitches were removed and the bandage was no longer required.

TIPS & ACTION ITEMS

- Hang a caddy below the shower mount (for shampoo, conditioner, liquid soap, etc.)
- Hang two scrubbies from the caddy (one should be blue. Blue for bum)
- Install a hand-held showerhead
- Install shower bars
- Consider a shower seat for your tub
- Place a rubber, non-slip mat in the bottom of the shower or tub
- Hang a towel close to the shower
- Learn how to dry yourself
- Hang a shower cap and hair wrap on the towel bar next to the shower
- Have your caregiver assist with your showers until your balance is good and you are comfortable doing it alone
- Place a non-slip rug in front of the shower

Taking Care
Of Your Incision

One of the risks of any surgery is infection, and it occurs about one percent of the time.

It is usually around ten days after surgery that infections present themselves, and it is extremely important to take note of such symptoms and **contact your surgeon immediately if any of these signs develop** during your spine surgery recovery:

- Fever 101 degrees or higher

- Redness at the incision site

- Increasing pain

- Change in the amount, appearance, or odor of drainage

An infection can be an extremely serious matter. First, four to six courses of intravenous antibiotics are required.

Second, further surgery could be needed to clean out the infection. Third, if the infection becomes chronic, the metal hardware that was installed during surgery may need to be removed. These are some pretty big reasons to insure your incision is being properly cared for.

I was fortunate to have caregivers who were as concerned as I about preventing any type of infection and who followed the instructions that were provided.

Each day after my shower, I sat on the side of the bed as my daughter carefully removed the clear bandage. Fortunately, the nurse provided us with some extra bandages before we left the hospital. It was much easier if both my husband and daughter worked together to replace the bandage. One was able to keep the adhesive from sticking to itself while the other placed and smoothed it over the incision area.

I have an allergy to adhesive. When my skin became irritated, my daughter placed a small piece of gauze over the area, under the adhesive. This prevented the area from itching and becoming further irritated.

Each day when the bandage was changed, either my husband or daughter took a photo of the incision. This allowed us to track the healing process and do side-by-side comparisons to note any changes that could signify infection moving in.

When I looked at the first photo, the incision looked to be a foot long, with many black stitches, but it was only about seven inches long. This was quite long enough to scare me. Thinking about someone cutting me open, moving my muscles over to the side, sawing bone away to make room for my nerves, attaching metal plates next to my vertebrae, and screwing them into the bone with long screws is significantly intimidating

I tried not to think back to the surgery process or the amount of time it would take to recover. Instead, I concentrated on what I needed to do each day to take care of myself and make sure the incision did not get infected.

Take the necessary steps to prevent infection. It is extremely important to keep your bed linens clean. This means keeping people and pets out of your bed. It also means bathing daily, putting on clean garments, and changing your linens every day.

These are the instructions I received for caring for my incision. If you do not receive written instructions, ask for them. Follow the directions carefully.

- Do not touch the incision
- Wash your hands before and after changing the dressing
- Keep the rest of your body clean
- Follow the instructions for using antibiotic soap

- Do not let anything come in contact with the incision

- Protect the incision from falls

- Do not sit in a bath, hot tub, or pool until your doctor approves

- Have everyone wash his/her hands when entering your room

- Make sure no one looks at or touches your dressing without washing his/her hands

- Change into clean clothes every day

- Avoid tight clothing that could irritate the incision

- Do not allow pets on your bed or furniture

- CHANGE THE SHEETS DAILY (think white - white can be bleached)

Now that we have considered the importance of properly caring for your incision and how my caregivers diligently followed the instructions, let's talk about something else that can be quite an uncomfortable experience during spine surgery recovery - the toilet.

TIPS & ACTION ITEMS

- Look out for signs of infection
- Caregivers learn how to change the bandage
- Learn how to handle adhesive allergy
- Take photos of the incision to track progress
- Learn how to take care of your incision
- Do not let anyone enter your bed in street clothes
- Change sheets daily

Sandra Joines

Business
in the Bathroom

Okay! Here we go with that thing we avoid discussing. My greatest fear about the entire surgery process was that someone was going to have to wipe my bum. And, I am sure that there are others out there with that same fear. As it turned out, I did not have to be concerned about that in the least. I could have spent the time worrying about something else. I assure you, I found many more things that teased my mind and caused me great angst.

Toilet

The first thing that helped me minimize my number one worry was the simple replacement of the toilet with a higher one. I never thought a couple of extra inches would allow me to sit and stand with less back pain. We chose a Kohler with a low gallon-per-flush rating for less than

$200. This does not include a cost for installation. The good news is that we received a seventy-dollar rebate from our water department.

Coming home from the hospital to a higher toilet was great, but I cannot wait to tell you about my favorite friend of all: a Brondell bidet toilet seat. This thing cost about $400. The cost was a little steep, but it happened to be Mother's Day and my birthday, so my three children and husband chipped in and bought it for me as a gift. I am excited beyond belief that they did.

If you have the extra dollars, invest in the Brondell bidet toilet seat and have it installed before you get home from surgery. I promise that you will not be disappointed.

The seat itself has temperature settings that are controlled by the handy remote controller, which can be installed on the wall where you can reach it without worrying about **NO BLT**. There are separate adjustments for the front and the back that control the temperature, the location of the spray, and the pressure of the spray. This device has my *#1 favorite* rating. Definitely worth the $400 if you have it.

I understand, however, that replacing a toilet with a higher one is not always easy and purchasing a $400 toilet seat cuts into the budget, but there are other options to help make your recovery process a little easier.

There are inexpensive bidet attachments for toilets for as little as $39.99 that can be purchased at your local Home Depot.

Sliding seats with legs that fit right over the toilet are also a good option, and they will provide you with support if you use the arms for leverage. There are seat risers with removable arms, extenders that are placed under the toilet, and plain old safety rails that can be installed. If your bathroom is a distance from your bed, a freestanding potty chair might come in handy.

My body had a tendency to bend forward when I sat or stood from the toilet. In retrospect, having access to handles on each side of the toilet would have minimized this tendency.

Another way to assist with sitting, standing, and preventing falls would be to install safety bars on the wall near the toilet. This would be another big bang for the buck.

Note: Using your walker for support for sitting or standing is a definite NO.

Once you become used to your higher toilet, use caution when sitting on a lower one. A couple of inches or less is a long way down.

Personal Hygiene

Since we are already talking about this delicate subject, let's say it like it is. Unless you have arms like an orangutan, some areas of your body are impossible to reach when you have a stiff back and a body throbbing with pain. **NO BLT.**

In the spine class I attended, the nurse held up a pair of *kitchen tongs* and told us that they would be very useful. She did not tell us exactly how they would be useful. We used our imagination. Not one person asked *how*. So, like everyone else, I figured it out on my own.

I quickly discovered that there is actually a trick to loading the tongs. First, with the tongs closed, run two baby wipes through the holes in the bottom of the tongs. Second, open the tongs enough to pinch a couple more baby wipes. You might have to move the wipes around a little to completely cover the metal of the tongs.

I have told you the *how* and I promise I will not leave you to figure the *why* out for yourself. If I had to guess, however, I think most of you have narrowed in on this. For those of you have not, the loaded tongs are used to wipe your bum.

Discard the used wipes in a trash can that you keep right next to the toilet. Remember, baby wipes stop up toilets. And also remember, when you drop the wipes into the trash, do not reach your arm across your body. Use the arm closest to the trash can. No **BLT.**

Trust me on this. Because of the pain and stiffness in your back and your instructions for **NO BLT**, keeping up with personal hygiene on certain areas of your body will be difficult without assistance. Using tongs, in conjunction with a bidet or a squirt bottle filled with warm water, might keep this assistance from being performed by a caregiver.

Remember my mentioning the *alcohol* I kept next to the sink? Well, now you know why. It is easy to pour some alcohol over the metal tongs to sterilize them before storing them.

Speaking of storing the tongs, a towel rack lives within easy reach of my toilet. I kept the tongs conveniently hung on the rack, along with some baby wipes that I clipped to the rack with a hair clip. **NO BLT.**

Constipation

Since we are discussing the lower regions, let's venture a little further. Everybody poops. At least we hope we do. The last thing we want right after surgery is constipation.

Anesthesia puts your muscles to sleep for surgery. The agents used in anesthesia can slow down the movement of stools in the colon, affect its motility, and depress the central nervous system.

Also, potent narcotic painkillers can also cause constipation after surgery by decreasing the gastrointestinal tract's peristaltic activity that pushes food material forward.

It is easy to understand how the side effects from anesthesia and pain killers, along with lack of exercise, an insufficient amount of liquids, and being subjected to hospital food, can prevent the plumbing from operating effectively.

When we are in the hospital, we are given stool softeners and perhaps mild laxatives. Then we are told to continue taking them when we get home. However, stool softeners do not have positive results for everyone. They tend to make the stool pasty, and this consistency is often times more difficult to expel than hard stools.

When you visit your primary care physician for your pre-op appointment have a conversation with her regarding what would work best for you. Should you start a Miralax regimen before surgery and continue it afterwards? Is it okay to take Milk of Magnesia to move things along after surgery? How frequently? Are suppositories or a Fleet enema options?

Eat foods that are high in fiber like veggies, fruit, and whole grain cereals. Drink lots of non-caffeinated beverages. Add prunes and prune juice as snacks. Sunkist has prunes with lemon or orange zest that are quite tasty. For me, the sure-fire remedy was fresh cherries.

And by all means, have these items on hand before surgery. Being proactive could prevent a painful occurrence of constipation. Unnecessary straining could put your surgical wounds at risk, and a blockage could mean an embarrassing trip to the emergency room.

Don't forget to have something on hand to relieve inflammation and pain from hemorrhoids that can pop up after a bout with constipation.

Sitting and standing from a toilet can be painful after surgery, and there can be a considerable amount of pain caused by straining while sitting on the toilet. What used to be a simple task of personal cleaning can become an almost impossible process. You have to adjust by learning new techniques and by remembering that not only is your back sore from surgery, it is also stiff, and bending is not an option.

I am sharing what I have learned through a considerable amount of thinking, analyzing, and practicing by good old trial and error, so that you can learn from my experiences and make your own learning process a little easier by anticipating and practicing before surgery.

Under normal situations, you seldom give thought to the simple task of how to dress yourself. Sure, you spend a considerable amount of time choosing what you are going to wear, but you give little thought as to how you will put this clothing on your body. During your spine surgery recovery, though, the simple task of dressing will be difficult, causing you unnecessary stress and demanding that you find an innovative way to do the simplest things. It will be considerably less painful and less stressful to know some helpful techniques before surgery.

Let's move on to dressing.

TIPS & ACTION ITEMS

- Face your greatest fear about surgery
- Install higher toilets
- Consider a Brondell bidet toilet seat
- Consider bidet toilet seat attachments
- Consider toilet seat extensions
- Consider portable potty chairs
- Install safety bars on walls where they are needed
- Learn how to properly load and use kitchen tongs for personal hygiene
- Use alcohol to sterilize tongs
- Have a squirt bottle on hand to use for personal hygiene
- Clip tongs and baby wipes to a towel bar located near the toilet
- Prevent constipation

Do I Have to Get Dressed?

I Can't Put on my Shoes and Socks

NO BLT, remember. When I was visiting with my surgeon at the pre-surgery appointment, he was kind enough to go over some of the restrictions that would be placed on me after surgery. Now, this man is tall and lanky and his legs stretch from his chin to the floor. You get the picture. He demonstrated what movements would be considered acceptable for putting on socks and shoes by placing one of his legs over the other and easily reaching with, oh yes, his long arms and with **NO BLT.**

Now some folks can cross one leg over the other with little effort and end up in a position that would allow them to slip on a sock and shoe and then tie the shoelace without bending or twisting. However, many of us are not blessed with those long legs.

The simplest remedy for this dilemma is to purchase, in advance, a pair of comfortable shoes that are easy to slip the foot into, yet fit tightly enough to control any slipping on the heel. The shoes should also have some awesome slip-proof soles.

I tried on an incredible number of shoes before surgery, looking for that perfect pair. My choice was a pair of Skechers Relaxed Fit Bikers Pedestrian Slip-On Walking Shoes that were priced at $64. This particular shoe allowed me to place my foot easily into the shoe without using my hand. Once my foot was in, I wiggled it around until my heel followed. The shoe offered a cushy inside, great support, and a sole with tread like a snow tire.

If you need to wear athletic shoes or men's dress shoes, you can place your sock on the floor by your foot, get out a trusty reacher, all of which I named "Jack," slip your toes into the sock, and work the sock over your foot with the reacher. It will take practice, patience, and time, but you will get there.

A device called a sock aid is available at medical supply stores or on Amazon. It is a rigid device with two handles that holds your sock open while you ease your foot all the way into the toe of your sock. It then helps you pull the sock up evenly. Cost is relatively low at about $8 to $13. If

I wore socks every day, I would have invested in one of these clever items.

A long shoe horn is another great aid in helping you to slip your foot into a shoe. DSW and other shoe stores give them away. Free is good.

Now, let's tackle tying the shoe. I recommend calling some cheerful family member or even some grumpy person around your home for assistance. As an alternative, you could invest in some new shoes with those little Velcro fasteners. **NO BLT.**

Why did I name my reachers "Jack," you ask? If you are familiar with the author Lee Child, you are most likely acquainted with his character Jack Reacher. Child said his wife was the reason he named his character Reacher. While shopping in grocery stores with his wife, Child was often asked by little ladies to reach an item on a high shelf. He told his wife the only use he had in a grocery store was to be a "reacher."

Underwear and Pants

Well, grab old "Jack" again. While sitting on the side of your bed or at a chair, place your undies on the floor by your feet and use the reacher to arrange the undies where you can easily place your feet into the openings. Use the reacher to pull them up your legs, one leg and then the other, above the knees. Then, holding one side of the undies with the reacher, stand. You may need some further assistance from the device to pull them up, but if you have long arms or raised the undies high enough on your thighs before you stood, you may be able to pull them up the remainder of the way with your own hands. Be sure to maintain your balance while you are pulling up your undies and resist the urge to reach across your body with your arm to pull up the opposite side.

This same procedure can be used for putting on pants. For a while after surgery, simple sweat pants with adjustable waist bands help keep unwanted pressure and rubbing away from your incision area.

Shaving

Unless you are a speedy healer and handle meds particularly well, shaving will most likely not be high on your list. Hopefully, you have a kind, generous person who hangs out around your house who is willing do this for you, or at least hand you an electric razor you can use while lying in bed watching imaginary critters crawl up and down your wall.

When you ladies get to a point where inch-long hairs on your legs begin to bother you, there is a way to hit most of the areas on your legs by yourself, without bending or twisting.

While lying on your back in your comfortable bed, you should be able to manipulate your legs into positions that allow you to cover almost all areas of your legs with an electric razor. This will be easier for some women depending on body type, flexibility, and the type of spine surgery performed.

The areas you are unable to reach will require the assistance of one of the kind, generous partners or friends to whom I have previously referred. Ladies, please make sure that while you are moving your legs and arms around, you do not bend or twist while trying to reach across your body. The person who changes your bed linen will appreciate your putting a towel under your legs to prevent those tiny hairs from taking up residence on the sheet. **NO BLT.**

Body Lotion – The Cricket Technique

This is one of my favorite tips. If you live in a dry climate or otherwise want to use lotion on your body, hopefully, there is someone around willing to apply this for you. If not, I discovered a way to reach almost every inch of my lower legs and most of my upper, without soliciting the help of old "Jack" or a caregiver.

While sitting on the edge of the bed, place a towel at your feet to protect the carpet or prevent tile or wood floors from becoming slippery. Use a reacher to move the towel around until it is directly under your feet.

The consistency of the product is important. Cream stays in place, allowing time to smooth it onto your legs. The best product I have found is Queen Helene Cocoa Butter

Face + Body Crème. It is the perfect consistency, does not have a loud smell, and I like the way it stays on the body. Try Rite Aid or Target for around $5.99 for fifteen ounces. It can also be ordered on Amazon.

Place a dollop of cream halfway between the knee and ankle, a little to the inside of the shin bone on your right leg. Using your left foot and leg, rub the cream onto your right leg, first using the bottom of your left foot, moving cream down the inside of your leg onto the top of the right foot and toes. Twist your foot around until the cream is rubbed into the back of the right leg with the top of your left foot. Your left toes should reach around to the outside of your right leg.

Get the picture? You simply use your left leg and foot - however it works best for you, to cover your right foot and leg with cream.

Now, switch legs. Place a dollop of cream on the same shin area of your left leg and then smooth it into your skin, with your right foot and leg, using the same motions.

By using your legs and feet, you can hit the backs and fronts of each lower leg as well as the bottom and top of each foot. It will be easy to find your own technique and rhythm. Your knees and the front of your thighs can be accessed by your hands, but you may have to be a little more creative to reach the back of your thighs. Think of a cricket rubbing his legs together.

It will be gratifying when you start feeling like doing more for yourself. This is the time when you begin to feel almost human again. You will be able to dress yourself and even apply body lotion using the *cricket technique.* And, perhaps, there will be other responsibilities you can take off the hands of your caregivers.

TIPS & ACTION ITEMS

- Purchase comfortable, slip-on shoes

- Consider shoes with Velcro fasteners

- Learn how to use a reacher to put on your socks

- Learn how to use a sock aid

- Learn to use a reacher to help put on undies and pants

- Purchase an electric razor

- Learn how to shave your legs with **NO BLT**

- Learn how to lather cream on your legs using the Cricket Technique

Sandra Joines

Laundry on a Leash

Now wait a minute! You don't really think you are going to get by with some generous person who loves you very much doing your laundry for the rest of your life. Besides, as you begin to feel better, you will actually want to do more for yourself, saving the more difficult things for your caregiver.

The day will come when someone is no longer taking care of your laundry, and you will need to find a way to take care of this task with **NO BLT.** There is a simple way to make this happen. Have someone run a belt through the handle of your laundry basket, and then pull the end of the belt through the buckle to make a leash. Or, use a dog leash.

If you have stairs to face like I do (you know, the Mount Everest type) it is easy to choke up on the leash, causing the clothes basket to stay close to your body. It will obediently follow you down, one step at a time.

Upon reaching solid ground, let out on the leash and pull the basket behind you.

And none other than the famous reacher will assist you with lifting the clothes from the basket (one piece at a time) and sorting them into piles before using the reacher to pick them up and place them into the washing machine.

When the laundry is ready for the dryer, again the reacher will allow you to remove the wet clothes from the washer and place them into the dryer. And yet again, use the reacher to remove the clothes from the dryer and place them into your clothes basket or hang them. From there you can pull the basket, by the leash, to your dining table. While sitting, it will be convenient for you to pick up a piece of clothing from the basket, using the reacher, and fold it on the table. Piece of cake, right?

We have discussed how something as simple as a belt can be the difference in your being able to take care of laundry or not. Let's look at some other devices that can significantly assist with your healing process and your mobility.

TIPS & ACTION ITEMS

- Learn to maneuver a laundry basket with **NO BLT**
- Use a reacher to move clothes to and from the washer and dryer

Sandra Joines

Helpful Devices

We have previously discussed some simple devices that can make your life easier during spine surgery recovery. There are other devices that may or may not be prescribed by your surgeon that could further facilitate your rehabilitation, as well as ones that can make a difference in your mobility.

Back Braces

Some surgeons require back braces for their spine surgery patients, while other surgeons leave the decision to wear one up to the patient. Discussing this during your pre-op surgery appointment is the perfect time to find out what your surgeon requires or recommends.

I was fitted with a brace at the pre-op appointment with my surgeon and was instructed to take it with me to the hospital. The hospital staff required me to wear it any time I was out of the bed.

Wearing the brace after returning home reminded me not to bend or twist and made me feel more secure.

Walker

During spine surgery class, I was informed that a walker would be waiting for me in the room I would be assigned to after surgery. I was required to use it, along with the back brace, each time I stood or walked. I came to the conclusion the first time I made a trip to the bathroom that the walker was an excellent idea. My walker, that I named "Johnnie," became my best friend.

Oxygen

Depending on your particular situation, you may be sent home from the hospital with oxygen. I was advised by a nurse that most patients who live in Colorado are sent home with oxygen due to the lower level of oxygen in the air because of the high altitude. Certain pain medications and medical conditions can also cause decreased oxygen levels, requiring the use of oxygen. **Follow your medical professional's advice.**

Cane or Walking Stick

I found a cane allowed me to move around a room without depending entirely on the bulky walker. When I was able to get out more, it helped me with balance, particularly in crowded situations. I also found the handle to be an invaluable tool to assist me in closing the car door. And, besides, I felt a bit safer having it in my possession. I reckoned if some character came along who wanted to take advantage of an old lady, I could inflict some hurt on him with the cane.

Portable Bone Stimulator

Electrical bone stimulators are a supplemental type of therapy that helps enhance the bone healing process and may or may not be prescribed by your surgeon. I had no idea that our body creates an electrical field that promotes the healing process. The bone stimulator helps the body's natural healing process by adding electrical current where it is needed.

This strange-looking device is connected to a belt that wraps around the waist and is secured with a Velcro fastener. It looks like a steering wheel from a race car and is worn for thirty minutes at the same time each day.

Rollator

The silver walker, "Johnnie," worked well around the house. However, after being advised by my surgeon to walk one or two miles a day, I discovered I could meet this requirement only with the assistance of a Rollator. On Amazon, I located a red Rollator with a basket, brakes, and a seat for an unbelievable low price of $48. You can also check out whether or not your insurance will cover this device.

This particular one weighed more than my limit for lifting, which made it necessary for someone else to remove it and return it to the trunk. A lighter weight Rollator can be purchased for a greater dollar amount.

Since the leg pain I was experiencing before surgery had not yet subsided, this device allowed me to walk with less pain, and the seat came in handy if I needed to rest for a spell. This is a huge bang for a small price.

As devices, like the ones mentioned above, are paramount in assisting in your healing process and your ability to be more mobile and independent during spine surgery recovery, the correct meds are also necessary to help you through your pain and healing. In the next chapter, let's look at meds and the role they play in the healing process.

TIPS & ACTION ITEMS

- Learn when to use back braces
- Learn about the importance of walkers
- Learn about the convenience of rollators
- Learn about the uses of canes or hiking poles
- Learn about using oxygen
- Learn about portable bone stimulators

Meds - the Good, Bad, and the Ugly

Your surgeon will put you on a pain medication regimen to help you get through the rough part of your spine surgery recovery. It is important to take the medication at the prescribed time even if you feel your pain is not strong enough to require it. Taking it as prescribed will help prevent you from having a difficult bout with pain and being required to take much stronger narcotics to calm it down. **ALWAYS FOLLOW YOUR PHYSICIAN'S INSTRUCTIONS ON HOW TO TAKE YOUR PAIN MEDS.**

Since pain meds cause nausea in some patients, you may be sent home from the hospital with a prescription for medication to prevent this. You may also have a prescription to help prevent muscle spasms. There may be other prescriptions, as well, based on your particular medical needs.

It is not unusual to experience side effects or allergic reactions to various types of pain medication, and this should not be taken lightly. I am one who experiences allergic reactions to every type of pain med I have been prescribed. It was no different during this journey.

Be confident about calling the doctor's office and asking for help. My physicians and other medical staff members were extremely speedy in switching the meds in order to find one that sufficiently reduced my pain without adding additional side effects. It wasn't, however, until I was able to tolerate pain by taking a small dosage of Norco at bedtime that the unpleasant side effects were reduced.

Most of the pain meds caused me to hallucinate. I saw words and images leaping from my iPad and attacking me, as well as bugs crawling on the wall. I experienced cold sweats and nausea. My stomach cramped. I felt loopy, dizzy, and drowsy, and I had to tolerate a constant headache. Then there was the heart that seemed to want to beat out of my chest and the body that resisted sleep. No, that's not all. My mouth was constantly dry, and food tasted terrible. My vision was blurred, and light bothered my eyes. I think the worst thing of all was the breaking out in hives and itching.

A list of medications that might be included in your pain management program and the side effects you could possibly experience should be provided to you by your physician or other medical professional. **While you are on these medications, do not stop them or change the**

dosage without the consent of your health professional. Do not drive. Do not drink.

CONSULT your physician to find out what symptoms are normal reactions caused by pain meds and which ones are immediate red flags.

If you experience any of the following symptoms, call your doctor or emergency room immediately:

- Extreme drowsiness

- Lightheadedness when changing positions

- Swelling of the face, tongue, or throat

- Feeling faint

- Trouble breathing

- Shortness of breath

- Chest pain

In the next chapter, let's discuss some of the nasty little things that can pop up at different times during your spine surgery recovery. Some are actually caused from certain medications you might be taking.

TIPS & ACTION ITEMS

- Types of meds
- What side effects to look for
- When to call the doctor
- When to call the emergency room
- Do not change or stop any meds without the direction of your doctor
- Normal reactions vs. red flags

Things That Pop Up

After spine surgery, there are **always** unexpected things that seem to suddenly present their ugly little heads. I seem to be a poster child representing those unexpected occurrences. You know, the picture with the verbiage, *if something is going to happen, it's going to happen to her*. That's me. I'll share a few of those with you.

Tooth Abscess

Sure enough, two weeks out from my surgery, I began to feel a throbbing pain in my lower left jaw. I concluded that it was from a tooth on which a root canal had been performed about three years prior. I immediately called the endodontist who had performed the procedure, and fortunately they were able to get me in that day.

I began thinking about no **BLT** and wondered how I would get my body into the dentist's chair without either bending or twisting. I shot an email to my surgeon's assistant, explaining the tooth situation, and asked how I could get onto the chair without breaking the golden rule of **NO BLT**. She immediately phoned back and advised me to log roll to the extent I could, **BUT under no circumstances** could any invasive procedure be performed.

WHAT?

She explained that if the infected area was compromised, the infection from the abscess could travel through my bloodstream and actually cause infection in the surgery area. I was almost knocked off my feet when she said this could ultimately cause meningitis. How was I to know this?

Why wasn't I told this by someone in the spine class, or by the doctor, or by the nurses in the hospital? Would it not be beneficial for spine surgery patients to be informed before surgery or before being released from the hospital? How many more things did I not know that I would be compelled to find out for myself? Okay. I know. They can't tell us everything. And, as my surgeon said, patients forget at least twenty percent of what they are told.

The endodontist took an x-ray, prescribed an antibiotic, and advised me that the pain meds I was taking should hold the pain down until the antibiotic had a chance to do its job.

It took about three days for the pain and throbbing to subside and the swelling to go down. I lived through those three days with an ice pack on my jaw and little relief from the Tylenol.

Yeast Infection

Now if you are a female, you understand what antibiotics can do to your body. Yep, that's right: *yeast infection*. One more thing added to my list of discomforts. I would highly recommend that all of you ladies have yeast infection treatment on hand. This is one of those just-in-case precautions. Better safe than sorry.

Thrush

Okay, since we are discussing yeast infections, another nasty result from antibiotics can be a good case of thrush. Yep, like the babies get. And, yes, the poster child was blessed with this also.

Dealing with crazy reactions from pain meds, experiencing some uncomfortable constipation (which resulted in uninvited hemorrhoids), a bout with thrush, and coping with extra pain and discomfort from an abscessed tooth were not enough.

Blood Clot

About a month after surgery, I was finally feeling a little chipper and decided to look over the user manual for a serger machine I had received for my birthday. My husband had recently begun feeling comfortable enough to leave me for a short time while he worked out. He had returned home from the health club, taken a shower, and was attending to some housekeeping downstairs. I was sitting in a comfortable office chair at my sewing table trying to determine if I would ever learn the ins and outs of this complicated machine or if it would sit on my sewing table gathering dust for the rest of its life and mine.

I was feeling pretty good for a change. Suddenly, however, I began to feel a strange sensation in my chest, as if something was crawling around. Pain began to replace this crawling sensation, making my chest feel full. As the pain traveled up my chest and into my neck and shoulders and as my heart began to race, I was certain an elephant was sitting on me. And then it hit me. I was having a heart attack, and I had gone through all this surgery pain and discomfort for nothing because I would no longer be here to know whether or not the surgery was a success.

After calling out to my husband, the next thing of which I was aware was lying on the floor, observing my husband on the phone with emergency personnel. He thought I had fallen out of the chair, and he was following hospital personnel's instructions to call 911 if I happened to fall.

He had been advised that only trained professionals should be allowed to lift me from the floor.

I was coherent enough to advise him that I had fallen from the chair because I had blacked out and to tell him what symptoms I had before I lost consciousness.

It took no time at all before five first responders were at my side, checking my vitals, and asking questions. They were extremely efficient and compassionate. Instead of worrying about my status, I was thinking how handsome these young men were and how much they reminded me of Chippendales. Not a thought was I giving to the poor old serger. Oh well! Call me a dirty old woman. But, if you ever have the need for first responders, think how nice it would be if they looked like these young men.

The good news is that I did not have a heart attack. It turned out to be a pulmonary embolism, which is the sudden blockage of a major blood vessel in the lung. In most cases, it is caused by a blood clot in the leg that breaks loose and travels to the lungs.

I consider myself blessed beyond belief. The fast action of my husband, the quick response from the first responders, and the efficient and speedy treatment from the emergency room medical staff prevented a more serious outcome. After a CT scan and other tests confirmed that my symptoms were caused by a blood clot, the nurse started an intravenous anticoagulant called Heparin. I continued to receive dosages of this medication until the next evening when I was discharged. I was prescribed an oral blood thinner called Xarelto and instructed to stay on oxygen twenty-four hours a day until further notice. I am required to take Xarelto for one year to keep my blood thin and to help prevent future blood clots.

You read earlier that this book is not about me or my surgery, but about you and what you can learn from my experiences. This is one of those experiences that I hope will make you aware of the rare possibility of blood clots happening and keep you alert to certain warning signs.

The Mayo Clinic advises us to contact a doctor if we experience swelling, redness, numbness, or pain in an area on a leg or an arm. And I think these signs are particularly difficult to separate from those symptoms we are already experiencing after having surgery. Please be aware. It is important to keep in mind that something of this nature can happen to you.

Mayo also advises us to reach out immediately for emergency attention if we experience any of these signs:

- Shortness of breath
- Pressure, fullness, or a squeezing pain in the center of your chest
- Pain extending to your shoulder, arm, back, or jaw
- A fast heartbeat
- Sudden weakness or numbness of your face, arm, or leg

- Sudden difficulty speaking or understanding speech
- Sudden blurred, double, or decreased vision

I have no idea if I experienced the last three symptoms because I passed out after the first four.

Discuss this possibility with your surgeon before surgery and ask him what you should look out for. Always consult your surgeon or other medical professional for instructions.

The day after I was released from the hospital, the old tooth abscess popped its ugly head once again. I was instructed to resume a regimen of antibiotics, Tylenol, and an ice pack.

Hair Loss

Although not life threatening, discovering clumps of hair in my hand while shampooing was rather frightening. I also began to notice that my brush was full of hair and there was an unusual amount of hair in my bed and on the floor.

The Mayo Clinic states that generalized loss of hair is usually due to one of the following: family history (heredity), hormonal changes, medical conditions, medications, or a major physical or emotional shock (surgery).

I would say that spine surgery would fall into the category of a major physical and emotional shock, and I have definitely had my share of different medications. Really? Is losing a third of my hair after everything else that has happened right? Of course not. But, it has happened, and I will deal with it. Besides, cute hats go a long way in taking care of bad hair days.

Unexpected things do pop up. There are numerous things you cannot prevent from happening, but you can prevent some things from being life threatening events by staying closely in touch with your body, by being aware of the type and degree of pain you normally endure, and by keeping your mind alert for anything that feels different.

TIPS & ACTION ITEMS

- Tooth Abscess
- Risks of dental work during recovery
- Yeast Infections
- Hemorrhoids
- Thrush
- Blood Clot
- Signs of blood clot
- Hair Loss
- Smell
- Taste

Let's Get Out
Of This House

At some point you will begin to feel more human and ready to venture out on outings that require getting in and out of vehicles. The more often you get in and out of vehicles, the faster you will develop your own technique and the easier it will become.

Getting In and Out of a Vehicle

If you are fortunate enough to have a vehicle with adequate headroom at the door, you will be able to back up to the seat and sit down without being concerned about manipulating your head. If you have lower headroom, however, you will have to find a way to duck your head under the door frame in such a way as to avoid bending or twisting.

Make sure there is a piece of plastic in the seat. A plastic shopping bag will work fine to help your body slide better as you turn to get yourself into and out of the vehicle. I found sitting back as far as I could when initially entering the car made the head issue less of a problem. Once you are sitting, place your left hand on the door frame and, while lifting your legs, turn slightly, moving both of your legs into the car and at the same time moving your left hand to a position on the dash, with your right arm following to a comfortable position. This should be one fluid movement and should be performed without bending or twisting. Watch the left hand to make sure that you do not try to extend it too far away from your body. Avoid trying to place your left foot into the vehicle and then moving the rest of your body in.

Once your body is in the car, work your left hand onto the console while at the same time moving your body to better face forward. The plastic bag will enable your body to easily slide over the seat. Using your left hand for support, push on the console and guide your body to a comfortable, even position. You will be tempted to move your left hand too far from your body, which will cause you to twist if you are not careful.

When exiting the car, use the directions in reverse.

Navigating Among People

Not only will you be slow getting in and out of the vehicle, you will also be slower than most of the people in stores who are rushing by you. Pay them no mind. You are not in their way. They can go around you. Making use of your walker or a cane when you are in crowds will allow you to navigate with less chance of your being thrown off balance by a passerby.

If the walker has brakes, engage them when you stop. And stop when you need to rest. If the walker has a seat, use it to rest from time to time. Always stop before you are exhausted. And ask for help when you need it. I find most strangers to be kind and most eager to help.

Your surgeon will advise you at what point you can drive. For me, it was after my three-month post-op visit. It was the first big sign for me that I would survive the recovery, and soon my requirement for assistance from someone else would be no longer an issue. I felt freedom knocking at my door.

TIPS & ACTION ITEMS

- How to get in and out of a vehicle
- How to be careful in crowds
- How to use a walker and cane for balance
- Don't overdo it
- Ask for help
- When you can drive

Wrapping It Up

Spine surgery is definitely not for the faint of heart. It is a complicated, intense procedure, and I have all the respect in the world for those people who choose to make surgery their profession. Our bodies, as well as our lives, are placed in their hands, and we trust that the outcome is worth the mental anguish and physical discomfort we are forced to endure.

Surgery is not only painful, debilitating, frustrating, confining, and overwhelming for patients, it also places a heavy burden on the families and caregivers. They hurt for us at times and feel inadequate to take care of us. Our inability to perform simple tasks requires us to rely on these caregivers, making us experience more stress.

There were times when I wanted to scream (and I did). There were other times when I simply wanted to cry (and I did). I desired being alone, with no sounds, no light, and certainly no voices from another human being. I despised being dependant on others and detested not being able to sit and stand without pain, or even lie in bed without pain.

Being connected to oxygen was confining, and using a walker and a cane became annoying. The back brace reminded me of **NO BLT**, but was restrictive. I felt trapped.

I did everything I was told, even if I did not fully understand it.

Before surgery, my surgeon told me that I would hate him for the first three months. He was right. There were days I did hate him, and everyone else for that matter.

Three months after surgery, I began to feel a little different. I noticed my pain level was not as high. And even though I was still unable to bend at my waist, I began to feel a tiny bit more limber, and walking was not as difficult. That was when I realized my body had once again agreed to cooperate with my mind, and I felt there was hope for a less painful life.

After the six-month point, learning to live with my restrictions was still a challenge, but the pain was less and moving and bending continued to improve.

The weeks keep ticking by. Each day I feel stronger and anticipate that I will continue to improve and live a less-painful life than I did before surgery. I try to concentrate on what I can do instead of what I can't.

I do not want to see my surgeon again. That could possibly mean additional surgery, and the thought of that sends out signals from every part of my body screaming, "NO NO

NO!" I will diligently follow his instructions for taking care of my back for the rest of my life.

I will also follow the exercise program provided to me by my brilliant physical therapist. It is up to me to keep my body strong and flexible by making the appropriate exercise program a part of my daily routine. It is up to me to maintain a healthy diet and keep hydrated by drinking an adequate amount of water. It is up to me to maintain an upbeat mental attitude and enjoy life to the fullest. I must be the person I am meant to be. I am responsible for my body and my life.

By sharing my experiences, I sincerely hope you will have a better understanding of how important it is to be a part of your medical decisions and to always be in charge of your body. Be proactive in choosing the best surgeon for you and your specific surgery. By all means, keep communication open among you and your surgeon, primary care physician, your caregivers, and any medical professional involved in your spine surgery recovery. Do not be afraid to ask any question, even if you think it might be unimportant to your medical professionals. Believe me, they have been asked every question you can imagine, and their job is to take care of your medical needs.

You can see that the suggestions I have shared are not complicated to implement and some cost absolutely nothing. If you choose to implement only a few of my ideas for preparing your home for your spine surgery recovery or follow a few of the instructions for taking care of yourself personally, I know you will find your life, as well as your caregivers' lives, considerably less stressful and painful.

Remember, any movement you can minimize will cause you less pain. And less pain means less stress. It's that simple.

Best of luck to you. Remember: follow the instructions provided by your surgeon and primary care physicians, follow the exercise plan your physical therapist has provided you, and stay in tune with your body during your healing process. You are in control of your body.

About The Author

Sandra Joines grew up and lived along the Gulf Coast of Florida before moving to Colorado. Being retired has provided her more time to spend with her family, write fiction, and enjoy the great outdoor activities Colorado affords. Well, until cycling, hiking, and kayaking came to a screeching halt due to her back issues and her ultimately being required to undergo a pretty nasty spine surgery.

She has turned the negative aspects of the physical pain, mental stress, inconvenience, and just plain agitation the surgery caused into an overwhelming desire to share what she has learned through her experiences with others who are facing or have had similar surgery.

You can learn more about Sandra at
www.SandraJoinesbooks.com.

Made in United States
Troutdale, OR
08/02/2023

11774817R00056